30minute solution Crohn's disease diet cookbook: for beginners

Just 30minite easy and fast delicious recipes to cute Crohn's pain, + special flavourful 28day meal plan to balance and stay healthy.

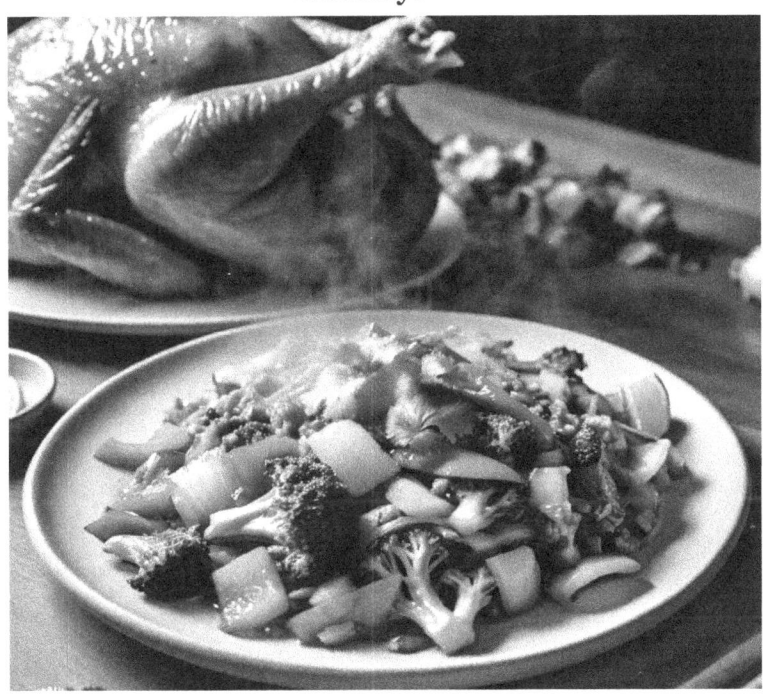

Dr. Jerry Cole

Copyright © 2024 Dr. Jerry Cole
Allright Reserved

No part of this publication may be reproduce, stored in a retrieval system, or transmitted in any form or by any means, electronic, mechanical, photocopying, recording or otherwise, without the prior permission of the copyright owner.

TABLE OF CONTENT

INTRODUCTION.. 6
WHAT ILLNESS IS CROHN'S?.. 7
COMPREHENDING CROHN'S DISEASE AND
DIGESTIVE HEALTH.. 9
NUTRITIONAL REQUIREMENTS AND DIETARY
CONSIDERATIONS... 12
IDENTIFYING TRIGGER FOODS..................................... 16
SPECIFIC DIETS FOR CROHN'S MANAGEMENT..... 19
SUPPLEMENTS AND SUPPORT FOR NUTRITION.. 23
HYDRATION AND FLUID INTAKE.................................. 27
SOCIAL SITUATIONS AND EATING OUT.................... 31
CONTROLLING WEIGHT AND APPETITE.................. 35
FOOD TO AVOID IN CROHN'S ILLNESS..................... 39
FOODS TO INCLUDE IN CROHN'S ILLNESS............. 43
COOKING FOR NOVICES WITH CROHN'S ILLNESS... 46
MEAL PLANNING AND RECIPES IN CROHN'S
DISEASE... 50
BREAKFAST RECIPES... 55
Banana Oatmeal Smoothie... 55
Scrambled Eggs with Spinach....................................... 56
Yogurt Parfait with Berries.. 57
Peanut Butter Banana Toast.. 58
Rice Porridge with Cinnamon and Applesauce....... 59
LUNCH RECIPES.. 60
Baked Chicken and Mashed Potatoes....................... 60
Quinoa Salad with Cucumber and Tomato.............. 62
Turkey and Cheese Wrap... 63

Salmon and Avocado Salad..64
Vegetable Stir-Fry with Rice....................................... 66
DINNER RECIPES... 67
Baked Salmon with Steamed Vegetables.................67
Turkey and Vegetable Stir-Fry................................... 69
Chicken and Rice Casserole..................................... 70
Spinach and Feta Stuffed Chicken Breast................ 71
Turkey and Rice Soup.. 73
DESSERT AND SNACK RECIPES............................. 75
Peanut Butter Banana Bites...................................... 75
Greek Yogurt with Honey and Berries...................... 77
Rice Cake with Almond Butter and Banana.............77
Trail Mix with Nuts and Dried Fruit........................... 78
Cottage Cheese with Pineapple Slices.....................79
APPETIZERS RECIPES... 80
Caprese Skewers... 80
Cucumber Hummus Bites..81
Greek Salad Skewers... 82
Stuffed Mini Bell Peppers.. 83
Smoked Salmon Cucumber Bites............................. 84
HEALTHY RECIPES... 85
Quinoa Salad with Lemon-Herb Dressing................85
Baked Chicken and Vegetables.................................87
Turkey and Quinoa Stuffed Peppers.........................89
Veggie and Bean Soup...90
Lentil Salad with Lemon-Tahini Dressing................ 92
28DAY MEAL PLAN... 94
Day 1:..94

Day 2: 95
Day 3: 97
Day 4: 98
Day 5: 99
Day 6: 100
Day 7: 101
Day 8: 102
Day 9: 103
Day 10: 104
Day 11: 104
Day 12: 105
Day 13: 105
Day 14: 106
Day 15: 107
Day 16: 107
Day 17: 108
Day 18: 109
Day 19: 109
Day 20: 110
Day 21: 110
Day 22: 111
Day 23: 112
Day 24: 112
Day 25: 113
Day 26: 113
Day 27: 114
Day 28: 115
CONCLUSION 115

THE END... 116

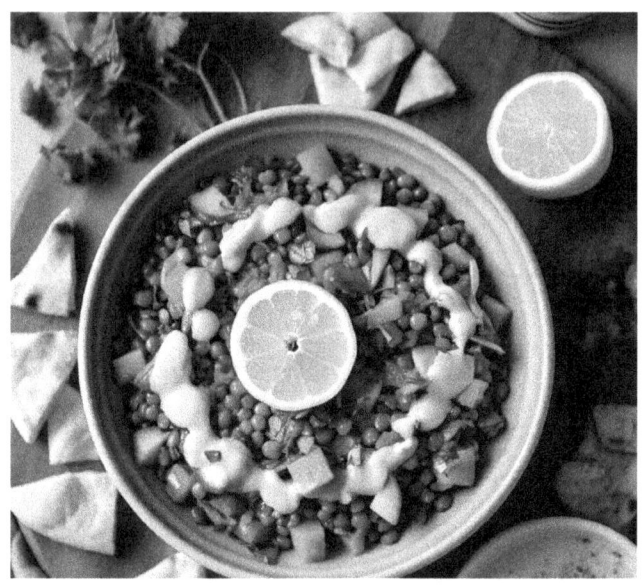

INTRODUCTION

"Welcome to the 30-Minute Solution Crohn's Disease Diet Cookbook for Beginners! If you're living with Crohn's disease, you know how challenging it can be to manage your symptoms and find delicious, easy-to-digest meals. But you're not alone! This cookbook is here to help you take control of your diet and your health, with quick, easy, and nutritious recipes that will make you feel good, not just okay.

In just 30 minutes a day, you can whip up a meal that will soothe your symptoms, satisfy your taste buds, and give you the energy to live your best life. Whether you're a busy bee or a culinary newbie, this cookbook is your perfect companion on the journey to healing and wellness. So let's get cooking, and let's take back control of our health, one delicious meal at a time!"

This introduction aims to:

- Welcome and reassure the reader that they're not alone in their struggles with Crohn's disease
- Emphasize the benefits of the cookbook: quick, easy, and nutritious recipes that will help manage symptoms and improve overall health

- Encourage the reader to take control of their diet and health
- End with a positive and uplifting note, inviting the reader to start their journey to healing and wellness.

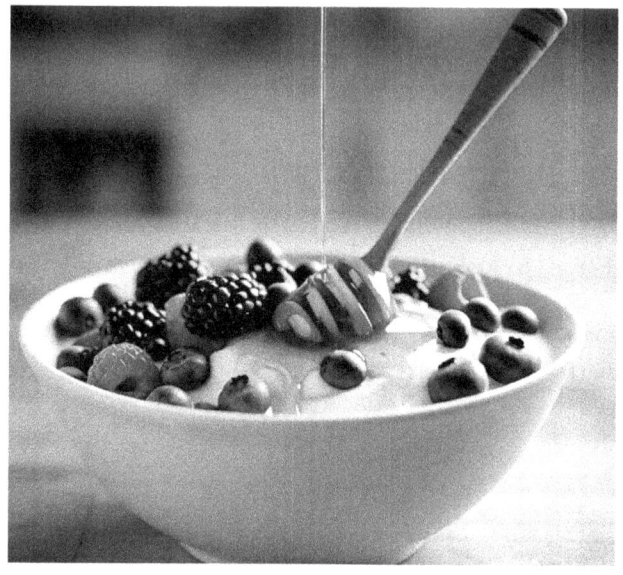

WHAT ILLNESS IS CROHN'S?

An inflammatory bowel disease (IBD) that mostly affects the gastrointestinal system is called Crohn's disease. It is a chronic condition. It can cause inflammation all the way from the mouth to the anus, although it usually affects the colon, which is the beginning of the large intestine, and the ileum, which is the end of the small intestine. Periods of flare-ups, when symptoms intensify, are typical in Crohn's disease. These are followed by periods of remission, when symptoms lessen or go away.

Crohn's disease symptoms can vary, but frequently include fever, exhaustion, diarrhea, and stomach pain. Severe cases may result in malnourishment, fistulas (abnormal connections between organs), and intestinal obstruction.

Although the precise origin of Crohn's disease is unknown, immune system, environmental, and genetic variables are thought to play a role. Although there is presently no known cure for Crohn's disease, patients can control their symptoms and enhance their quality of life with the use of medications, lifestyle modifications, and in certain situations, surgery.

COMPREHENDING CROHN'S DISEASE AND DIGESTIVE HEALTH

Comprehending the health of the digestive system is essential to effectively managing diseases such as Crohn's disease. Food digestion, nutrient absorption, and waste removal are all handled by the digestive system. When healthy cells in the digestive tract are wrongly attacked by the immune system, it results in Crohn's disease patients' inflammation and a variety of other symptoms.

Preserving optimal digestive health necessitates multiple crucial elements:

Nutrition: To maintain digestive health, a balanced diet full of fruits, vegetables, whole grains, lean meats, and healthy fats is recommended. Some Crohn's disease sufferers may need to stay away from foods like dairy, spicy foods, or meals high in fiber because they aggravate their symptoms. Creating a customized food plan might be facilitated by working with a dietician.

Hydration: Getting enough water into your system is crucial for healthy digestion and general wellbeing. Fatigue and diarrhea are two symptoms that might get worse from dehydration.

Stress management: Since stress can aggravate Crohn's disease symptoms, learning practical stress-reduction strategies like mindfulness, meditation, yoga, or regular exercise might be helpful.

medicine: Depending on the severity of the symptoms, medical professionals may recommend medicine to treat pain or diarrhea, lower inflammation, or suppress the immune system. It's critical to take prescription drugs as directed and to discuss any adverse effects or concerns with medical professionals.

Frequent Monitoring: It's critical to visit your doctor on a regular basis to monitor the progression of your illness, evaluate your nutritional state, and modify your treatment plan as necessary. Monitoring can assist in identifying any issues early on and shield the digestive system from long-term harm.

Lifestyle Modifications: Reducing weight, exercising frequently, and giving up smoking can all help improve gut health and general wellbeing.

Support System: Having a network of family, friends, and medical professionals who are there for you during difficult times can be quite beneficial when living with Crohn's disease. Online networks and support groups can also offer priceless information and assistance.

People with Crohn's disease can enhance their quality of life and better manage their illness by putting these gut health components first and collaborating closely with medical professionals.

NUTRITIONAL REQUIREMENTS AND DIETARY CONSIDERATIONS

Because Crohn's disease affects the digestive system, it is especially vital for those who have IBD to take dietary considerations and nutritional demands seriously. Here are some important things to think about:

Diet: Consuming a varied range of nutrients in a balanced diet is crucial for good general health. Fruits, vegetables, whole grains, lean meats, and good fats are all included in this. Maintaining a food journal can be beneficial for certain Crohn's disease sufferers in order to pinpoint trigger foods and improve their diet.

Low-Fiber Foods: People with Crohn's disease may find it helpful to eat easier-to-digest low-fiber foods during flare-ups. Tender meats, white bread, refined grains, and cooked or peeled fruits and vegetables may be examples of this.

High-Calorie and High-Protein Foods: People with Crohn's disease may worry about malnutrition and weight loss, particularly during flare-ups. Eating foods high in calories and protein can assist sustain energy levels and promote recovery. Nuts, seeds, nut butters, eggs, dairy (if tolerated), and lean meats are nutrient-dense foods.

Hydration: It's important to stay hydrated because Crohn's disease frequently causes diarrhea and dehydration. Dehydration can be avoided by drinking lots of water throughout the day and abstaining from alcoholic or caffeinated drinks.

Supplements: Inflammation or damage to the digestive tract can sometimes make it difficult for people with Crohn's disease to absorb certain nutrients. To treat deficiencies, supplements like calcium, iron, vitamin B12, vitamin D, and omega-3 fatty acids may be suggested.

Steer clear of Trigger Foods: People with Crohn's disease may have increased inflammation or symptoms from certain foods. Dairy, high-fiber diets, spicy foods, coffee, and alcohol are common triggers. Reducing flare-ups and managing symptoms can be achieved by identifying and avoiding trigger foods.

Small, Frequently Spaced Meals: Eating smaller, more spaced-out meals throughout the day will lessen the strain on the digestive tract and lessen symptoms like diarrhea, cramping, and bloating.

Consultation with a dietician: Seeking the advice and support of a licensed dietician with expertise in gastrointestinal issues can be beneficial. A dietitian can assist in developing a customized meal plan, addressing dietary deficits, and tracking dietary modifications over time.

All things considered, maintaining a well-balanced diet, drinking plenty of water, and attending to particular nutritional requirements might assist people with Crohn's disease better manage their illness and enhance their quality of life.

IDENTIFYING TRIGGER FOODS

Determining the foods that cause inflammation can be essential to controlling Crohn's disease and minimizing flare-ups. Although each person's trigger meals may be different, some typical ones are as follows:

High-Fiber Foods: Foods high in insoluble fiber can be hard to digest and can make symptoms like bloating, diarrhea, and stomach pain worse. Examples of such foods include fresh fruits and vegetables, whole grains, nuts, and seeds.

Dairy Products: Some people with Crohn's disease may experience issues with lactose-containing dairy products, such as milk, cheese, and yogurt, particularly if they are lactose intolerant. Making the switch to dairy-free or lactose-free options could be advantageous.

Spicy meals: For certain Crohn's disease sufferers, spicy meals can aggravate their digestive system and cause inflammation. Reducing or avoiding spicy foods, condiments, and sauces may help ease symptoms.

High-Fat dishes: Foods that are high in saturated and trans fats, like fried dishes, fatty meat cuts, and processed snacks, might be more difficult to digest and exacerbate symptoms like upset stomach and diarrhea.

Caffeine and Alcohol: For some people with Crohn's disease, caffeine and alcohol might stimulate the digestive tract, resulting in increased bowel motions and discomfort. Alcoholic and caffeinated drinks should be avoided or consumed in moderation to assist manage symptoms.

Raw Vegetables and Fruits: Although they are nutrient-dense, some Crohn's disease sufferers may find it difficult to digest fruits and vegetables in their raw state. Fruits and vegetables can be easier to tolerate if they are cooked or steamed.

Carbonated Drinks: People with Crohn's disease may experience discomfort due to gas and bloating from carbonated drinks, such as soda and sparkling water. It could be better to choose herbal teas or still water instead.

Artificial Sweeteners: Certain artificial sweeteners, like sorbitol and mannitol, can have a laxative effect and exacerbate Crohn's disease symptoms like gas and diarrhea.

Gluten: Although celiac disease is more frequently linked to gluten intolerance, certain Crohn's disease patients may also be sensitive to gluten-containing foods such wheat, barley, and rye. Those who are sensitive to gluten might find it beneficial to try a gluten-free diet.

Keeping a food journal is crucial for people with Crohn's disease in order to monitor their nutritional intake and any related symptoms. They can identify particular dietary triggers and make educated dietary selections to assist effectively manage their illness by gradually removing probable trigger items and monitoring how their bodies react. Seeking advice from a medical professional or registered dietitian can also offer tailored direction and assistance in determining trigger foods and implementing dietary adjustments.

SPECIFIC DIETS FOR CROHN'S MANAGEMENT

Numerous dietary strategies have been put out to manage Crohn's disease, albeit each person's reaction may differ. The following are some particular diets that people with Crohn's disease might think about:

The low-FODMAP diet involves consuming carbohydrates known as FODMAPs (fermentable oligosaccharides, disaccharides, monosaccharides, and polyols), which can ferment in the gut and result in symptoms such as gas, diarrhea, and bloating. In order to identify triggers, the low-FODMAP diet entails temporarily limiting intake of high-FODMAP foods and then gradually returning them. This strategy might benefit certain Crohn's disease patients with their gastrointestinal issues.

Specific Carbohydrate Diet (SCD): To lessen inflammation and encourage the healing of the digestive tract, the SCD prohibits a number of carbs, such as grains, sweets, and the majority of dairy products. Nutrient-dense foods are highlighted, including meats, seafood, eggs, fruits, vegetables, nuts, and some dairy products. Although there is little scientific evidence to support the usefulness of the SCD, some Crohn's disease patients experience relief in their symptoms.

Paleo Diet: The Paleo Diet excludes grains, dairy, legumes, and processed foods in favor of whole, unprocessed foods that were likely ingested by early humans, such as lean meats, fish, fruits, vegetables, nuts, and seeds. Although individual results can vary, some Crohn's disease patients may find symptom alleviation with the Paleo Diet.

Gluten-Free Diet: Although celiac disease is more frequently linked to gluten intolerance, Crohn's disease patients might also be sensitive to gluten-containing foods. Products made from wheat, barley, rye, and their derivatives are not allowed in a gluten-free diet. A gluten-free diet has been reported to help some Crohn's disease patients with their symptoms, but there isn't any scientific proof to support this treatment's efficacy for the condition in particular.

Anti-Inflammatory Diet: This type of diet emphasizes foods like fruits, vegetables, nuts, seeds, fatty fish, and good fats that can help lower inflammation in the body. Additionally, it restricts or stays away from meals like processed foods, refined carbohydrates, and trans fats that could exacerbate inflammation. Although there isn't a specialized anti-inflammatory diet for Crohn's disease, adhering to the broad guidelines of one could help control symptoms and promote general health.

When thinking about making dietary adjustments, people with Crohn's disease should collaborate closely with healthcare professionals, especially a licensed dietitian or nutritionist. These experts can offer tailored advice, keep an eye on nutritional status, and guarantee that dietary adjustments are suitable and safe for each person's requirements. Furthermore, even though dietary modifications could assist some people in managing their symptoms, they cannot replace medical care; prescription drugs from medical professionals are still a crucial part of managing Crohn's disease.

SUPPLEMENTS AND SUPPORT FOR NUTRITION

Supplements and nutritional assistance can be very helpful in treating nutrient deficiencies and promoting general health when it comes to controlling Crohn's disease. The following are important dietary concerns and supplements for people with Crohn's disease:

Multivitamin and Mineral Supplements: If the diet is restricted or malabsorption is a concern, a high-quality multivitamin and mineral supplement can assist fill in nutritional gaps and avoid deficiencies. Seek out supplements designed especially for those with digestive issues, as they might have more easily absorbed forms of certain nutrients.

Calcium and Vitamin D: Because of conditions like inflammation, malabsorption, and steroid use, people with Crohn's disease may be more susceptible to osteoporosis. Supplements containing calcium and vitamin D can assist maintain healthy bones. It's critical to collaborate with a healthcare professional to assess bone density over time and select the right dosage based on individual needs.

Omega-3 Fatty Acids: Rich in anti-inflammatory qualities, omega-3 fatty acids can help people with Crohn's disease feel less irritated. You can find them in fish oil supplements. For those who are unable to consistently eat fatty fish, fish oil supplements may be very helpful. Before beginning an omega-3 supplement regimen, it's crucial to speak with a healthcare professional as some drugs may interfere with omega-3 supplements.

Probiotics: Probiotics are good bacteria that can assist digestive health and help the gut microbiome rebalance. According to some study, some probiotic strains may help people with Crohn's disease experience better symptoms and less inflammation. Probiotic efficacy, however, can differ based on the strain and personal reaction. Selecting probiotic supplements that have been carefully researched for Crohn's disease is preferable, as is talking about supplementing with a medical professional.

Iron: People with Crohn's disease frequently have iron deficiency anemia, particularly if they are experiencing active inflammation or gastrointestinal bleeding. It could be required to take iron supplements to make up for any deficiencies and to relieve symptoms like weakness and exhaustion. A healthcare professional should regularly manage iron supplements since taking too much iron might have negative consequences on the gastrointestinal system.

B12 Injections: Due to inflammation or damage to the ileum, which is where B12 absorption takes place, some people with Crohn's disease may have trouble absorbing vitamin B12 from diet. B12 injections or oral supplements could be required in these situations in order to avoid deficits and neurological issues.

Enteral Nutrition: Enteral nutrition may be used as a primary or supplemental treatment in some circumstances, particularly in children with Crohn's disease. Enteral nutrition refers to the oral or feeding tube administration of a nutritionally complete liquid formula. It can stimulate growth and development, assist bring an illness into remission, and offer nourishment when symptoms flare again.

It is imperative that people with Crohn's disease speak with a healthcare physician, especially one with experience in gastroenterology or nutrition, before beginning any new supplements or dietary therapies. A medical professional may evaluate each patient's unique nutritional requirements, keep an eye out for any drug interactions, and make tailored suggestions for dietary supplements and support. Furthermore, depending on the disease activity, the response to treatment, and changes in nutritional status over time, continued monitoring and modifications can be required.

HYDRATION AND FLUID INTAKE

For those with Crohn's disease, maintaining adequate fluid intake and hydration is vital, particularly during flare-ups when symptoms like diarrhea can cause dehydration. The following are important things to remember:

Drink A Lot of Water: Remaining hydrated is important for general health and can help reduce dehydration-related symptoms like weariness and lightheadedness. Eight 8-ounce glasses of water should be consumed daily, while this number might vary depending on personal needs, activity level, and weather conditions.

Electrolyte Balance: Keeping your electrolyte balance is crucial, especially if you're throwing up or have diarrhea. You should also drink plenty of water. Electrolytes—such as sodium, potassium, and chloride—are necessary for healthy muscular contraction and fluid equilibrium. Electrolytes lost due to diarrhea can be replaced by ingesting electrolyte-rich foods and beverages such as sports drinks, coconut water, bananas, and broth, or by drinking oral rehydration treatments.

Watch Urine Color: The color of your urine can give you a good indication of how hydrated you are. Dark yellow urine may indicate dehydration, but clear or pale yellow pee usually suggests enough hydration. Aim for pale yellow urine to indicate that you are getting enough water.

Limit Alcohol and Caffeine: These substances have diuretic properties that can raise urine production and perhaps exacerbate dehydration. Drinking fewer or no alcoholic and caffeinated beverages can help you stay hydrated.

Fluid Intake Throughout the Day: Try to distribute your fluid intake throughout the day rather than consuming a lot of it all at once. Regularly consuming liquids, such as water, can assist maintain hydration and prevent dehydration.

Modify Fluid Intake During Flare-Ups: Higher fluid losses can occur during Crohn's disease flare-ups when symptoms like diarrhea are more acute. To counteract losses and keep hydrated during these periods, it could be essential to increase fluid intake. It could be required to receive intravenous (IV) fluids in a medical environment if dehydration is severe or chronic.

Be Aware of Oral Rehydration Solutions: During episodes of diarrhea or vomiting, oral rehydration solutions (ORS), such as Pedialyte or Gatorade, can be useful for restoring fluid and electrolyte balance. However, because ORS include certain components or have a high sugar level, some people with Crohn's disease may need to use them with caution. Safe use can be ensured by choosing adult-specific ORS formulations or by speaking with a healthcare professional.

Speak with a Healthcare Professional: It's crucial to talk to a healthcare professional if you have any concerns regarding electrolyte balance, fluid consumption, or hydration. They can offer tailored advice depending on your particular demands, medication schedule, and state of health.

People with Crohn's disease can better manage their symptoms, support their general health, and lower their risk of consequences from dehydration by prioritizing fluid intake and staying hydrated.

SOCIAL SITUATIONS AND EATING OUT

For people with Crohn's disease, going out to eat and navigating social settings can provide special obstacles. However, with some preparation and strategy, it is possible to enjoy social occasions while efficiently managing symptoms. The following advice will help you manage social situations and eat out when you have Crohn's disease:

Investigate Restaurants: Do some advance research on restaurants to identify those that will accommodate your dietary requirements and preferences before heading out to dine. Seek out eateries with a diverse menu that includes dishes that are likely to be well-tolerated and easily digested.

Call Ahead: To find out about menu alternatives and accommodations, give the restaurant a call in advance if you have any special dietary needs or preferences. By doing this, you can make sure the restaurant can meet your needs and alter the food as needed.

Ask Questions: Feel free to enquire about the preparation of dishes and whether specific components can be left out or replaced with others from your server. Dietary restrictions can usually be accommodated in restaurants, especially if they are communicated in advance.

Select Easy Preparations: Go for foods that are simple to prepare and quick to digest, like sautéed vegetables, basic rice or potatoes, and grilled or steamed proteins. Steer clear of foods that are fried, highly spiced, or have creamy dressings or rich sauces as they can make symptoms worse.

Portion Control: To prevent overeating, which can worsen symptoms like bloating and discomfort, pay attention to portion sizes and think about ordering smaller servings or sharing dishes with dining companions.

Bring Your Medications with You: If you take medication to help with Crohn's disease symptoms, make sure you bring them along when you eat out. In this manner, you'll be ready if, while traveling, you have symptoms or flare-ups.

Drink lots of water to stay hydrated when dining out. This is especially important if you're also having caffeinated or alcoholic beverages, which can dehydrate you.

Be Aware of Trigger Foods: When dining out, try to avoid or restrict trigger foods that might aggravate symptoms. Reading ingredient lists and enquiring about the preparation methods of dishes may be necessary for this.

Savor Social Interaction: Rather of concentrating only on the cuisine when dining out, try to enjoy the company of friends and family. Talk to each other, enjoy your meal, and value the chance to interact with others.

Listen to Your Body: Keep an eye on how your body reacts to various meals and dining situations, and modify as necessary. If particular meals or dining establishments frequently cause symptoms, you might want to steer clear of them going forward.

People with Crohn's disease can confidently manage social situations including eating out while managing their condition if they are proactive, knowledgeable, and flexible.

CONTROLLING WEIGHT AND APPETITE

Because Crohn's disease can impair digestion, weight control, and overall energy balance, these issues can be very important to those who have the illness. The following are some methods for controlling hunger and weight in people with Crohn's disease:

Nutrient-Dense Foods: To promote general health, make an effort to eat a diet high in vitamins, minerals, and calories. Pick foods like lean meats, fish, eggs, nuts, seeds, fruits, vegetables, and whole grains that are high in protein, healthy fats, and complex carbs.

Smaller, More Often Meals: Throughout the day, eating smaller, more often meals might help control symptoms including pain, bloating, and early satiety. This strategy can also aid in maintaining a consistent intake of calories and nutrients, even in cases where hunger is diminished.

Liquid and Soft Foods: Go for foods that are easily digested, such as soups, smoothies, yogurt, and pureed fruits and vegetables, during flare-ups or periods of decreased appetite. These choices might be easier to accept and easy on the digestive tract.

Keep an Eye on Portion Sizes: Overeating can aggravate symptoms like bloating, gas, and discomfort, so be mindful of portion sizes and avoid it. Reduce the size of your dishes and cutlery to help you manage portion sizes and avoid overindulging.

Drink lots of water to stay hydrated throughout the day. This will help you feel fuller and have more energy. Limit diuretic beverages like coffee and alcohol and opt instead for hydrating options like water, herbal tea, and broth.

Handle Stress: Since stress can have an impact on digestion and hunger, learning practical stress-reduction strategies such as mindfulness, yoga, meditation, or relaxation techniques might be helpful. Supporting appetite and general well-being can be achieved by making self-care a priority and learning constructive stress management techniques.

Consult a Dietitian: To create a customized food plan and nutritional approach, think about consulting a registered dietitian with expertise in gastrointestinal issues. A dietician can offer advice on controlling weight and appetite in people with Crohn's disease, as well as help identify trigger foods and vitamin deficits.

Supplements: To support nutritional status in cases of malnutrition or nutrient shortages, supplements may be required. See a doctor if you think you would benefit from taking supplements like protein powders, meal replacement drinks, or multivitamins.

Medication Management: Certain drugs, such corticosteroids, that are used to treat Crohn's disease can have an impact on weight and appetite. If you notice changes in your appetite or weight while taking medication, talk to your doctor about these issues.

Frequent Monitoring: Under the supervision of a healthcare professional, keep a close eye on your weight, appetite, and nutritional status. Regular evaluations can assist in spotting patterns or changes over time and help direct necessary dietary and therapeutic strategy changes.

People with Crohn's disease can improve general health and well-being while managing weight and appetite changes by using these techniques and collaborating closely with healthcare specialists.

FOOD TO AVOID IN CROHN'S ILLNESS

Certain foods can aggravate symptoms and cause flare-ups in people with Crohn's disease. Although each person's trigger foods may be different, the following are some typical ones to think about restricting or avoiding:

High-Fiber Foods: Foods high in fiber can exacerbate symptoms like diarrhea, bloating, and abdominal pain since they are difficult to digest. Examples of such foods include raw fruits and vegetables, whole grains, seeds, and nuts. Fruits and vegetables can be made easier to accept by steaming or cooking them, as well as by choosing refined grains.

Dairy Products: Milk, cheese, and yogurt might cause issues for certain people with Crohn's disease, as lactose intolerance is frequent in this population. Selecting dairy-free or lactose-free options might help lessen symptoms like diarrhea, bloating, and gas.

Spicy meals: For those with Crohn's disease, spicy meals may cause discomfort and inflammation by irritating the digestive system. Restricting or avoiding spicy foods, sauces, and spices may aid with symptom management.

dishes High in Saturated and Trans Fats: Foods that are high in these fats, like fried dishes, fatty meat cuts, processed snacks, and creamy sauces, can be more difficult to digest and aggravate symptoms like diarrhea and stomach pain.

Alcohol and Caffeine: In many Crohn's disease sufferers, alcohol and caffeine can aggravate symptoms such as diarrhea, urgency, and discomfort in the abdomen by stimulating the digestive system. Alcoholic and caffeinated drinks should be avoided or consumed in moderation to assist manage symptoms.

Carbonated Drinks: People with Crohn's disease may experience discomfort due to gas and bloating from carbonated drinks like soda and sparkling water. It could be better to choose still water or non-carbonated drinks.

High-Sugar Foods: Candy, candies, sweets, sugary drinks, and desserts are examples of foods and drinks with a lot of added sugar that can aggravate symptoms including diarrhea, bloating, and gas. Making the switch to lower-sugar options could aid with symptom management.

Processed and Spicy meals: Additives, preservatives, and spices are frequently included in processed meals like chips, crackers, fast food, and processed meats, which can make symptoms worse for those with Crohn's disease. It could be advantageous to select whole, minimally processed foods whenever feasible.

Foods containing gluten: Crohn's disease patients may also be sensitive to gluten, even though gluten intolerance is more frequently linked to the illness. If there is a suspicion of gluten sensitivity, foods containing wheat, barley, rye, and their derivatives should be restricted or avoided.

Raw Vegetables and Fruits: Although they are nutrient-dense, some Crohn's disease sufferers may find it difficult to digest fruits and vegetables in their raw state. Fruits and vegetables can be easier to tolerate if they are cooked or steamed.

It's crucial to remember that every person reacts differently to food, so keeping a food journal and monitoring how various meals impact symptoms may be beneficial. Speaking with a medical professional or registered dietitian can offer individualized advice on dietary adjustments and assist in identifying trigger foods that are unique to each person's requirements.

FOODS TO INCLUDE IN CROHN'S ILLNESS

Including nutrient-dense, easily digestible, and gentle on the digestive tract diets can help manage symptoms and promote overall health in those with Crohn's disease. The following items should be included in a diet that is Crohn's disease-friendly:

Lean Proteins: If you can stomach it, choose easily digested forms of lean protein including skinless chicken, fish, eggs, tofu, and lentils. These meals supply vital amino acids needed for general health and muscle regeneration.

Vegetables: In general, cooked or steamed veggies are simpler to stomach than their raw counterparts. Select cooked veggies that are high in vitamins, minerals, and fiber, such as green beans, potatoes, zucchini, squash, and carrots.

Ripe Fruits: Soft, easily chewed ripe fruits may be easier on the digestive system. Good choices that are high in vitamins, minerals, and fiber include bananas, applesauce, melons, peaches, and cooked fruits like apples and pears.

Pasta and White Rice: Both white rice and pasta are simple, readily absorbed carbs that can provide you energy without making your digestive problems worse. Steer clear of any potentially irritating sauces or seasonings and go for simple white rice or pasta.

Reduced-Fiber Grains: Choose reduced-fiber pasta, white bread, white rice, and refined cereals. These meals are less likely to aggravate symptoms like diarrhoea and cramping in the abdomen.

Good Fats: Include foods high in healthy fats, such as nuts, seeds, avocado, olive oil, and fatty fish, in your diet. In addition to offering important fatty acids, these fats can aid in satiety and the absorption of nutrients.

Dairy Alternatives: If lactose sensitivity is a concern, select lactose-free or dairy substitutes such as lactose-free cheese, yogurt, almond milk, and coconut milk. These solutions supply calcium and additional nutrients without compromising intestinal health.

Healthy Soups and Broths: Homemade bone broth, transparent vegetable broth, or pureed veggies can all be rich sources of nutrients and hydration while still being gentle on the digestive system.

Nut Butters: Packed with calories, protein, and good fats, nut butters such as almond, sunflower seed, and peanut butters are a quick and wholesome snack choice.

Hydration: Stay hydrated throughout the day by drinking lots of water, especially if you're throwing up or have diarrhea. Coconut water, herbal teas, and electrolyte-rich drinks are other drinks that can help rehydrate and avoid dehydration.

It's critical to pay attention to how different foods affect your symptoms and to your body's signals. Maintaining a food journal can assist in identifying trigger foods and customizing your diet to improve Crohn's disease management. Speaking with a medical professional or certified dietitian can offer individualized advice on dietary changes and guarantee that nutritional requirements are satisfied while successfully controlling symptoms.

COOKING FOR NOVICES WITH CROHN'S ILLNESS

Cooking with Crohn's disease can be intimidating at first, especially for newcomers, but it can be doable and even fun with a little preparation and easy techniques. Here are some pointers for first-time Crohn's disease cooks:

Start Simple: Start with dishes that are easy to make and call for few ingredients and preparation processes. Seek meals that feature foods that are simple to digest, such as prepared veggies, lean proteins, and low-fiber grains.

Emphasis on Fresh, Whole Foods: Try to eat as many fresh, whole foods as you can because they are generally easier to digest and have less additives and preservatives. To achieve balanced nutrition, include a range of fruits, vegetables, lean proteins, and healthy fats in your meals.

Cooking Techniques: Use cooking techniques like steaming, boiling, poaching, baking, or grilling that are easy on the digestive system. These techniques reduce additional fats and oils while preserving nutrition.

Portion Control: Be mindful of serving sizes to prevent overindulging, which can make symptoms like pain and bloating worse. Reduce the size of your dishes and cutlery to help you manage portion sizes and avoid overindulging.

Meal Planning: Arrange your meals and snacks ahead of time to guarantee a balanced diet and steer clear of impulsive decisions that can result in less nutrient-dense options. To save time and make meal preparation easier during the week, think about batch cooking and meal prep.

Gently Seasonings: Select spices and seasonings that aren't likely to aggravate the digestive system. Simple seasonings like salt and pepper, fresh herbs, and mild spices like ginger and turmeric can all provide taste without making symptoms worse.

Maintain a Food Diary: By keeping a food diary, you can monitor your diet and how it impacts your symptoms. Make a mental note of any items that appear to exacerbate symptoms or flare-ups so that you can make well-informed dietary choices.

Keep Yourself Hydrated: Stay hydrated by drinking lots of water throughout the day, especially if you're throwing up or have diarrhea. To rehydrate and avoid dehydration, choose hydrating drinks like water, herbal tea, and clear broths.

Listen to Your Body: Observe how certain foods impact your symptoms and modify your diet in response. If specific foods are known to cause symptoms on a regular basis, you may want to limit or avoid them going forward.

Seek Support: If you need advice or encouragement, don't be afraid to get in touch with medical professionals, licensed dietitians, or support groups. They can offer tailored guidance, dietary suggestions, and useful hints for controlling Crohn's disease with dietary and lifestyle adjustments.

People with Crohn's disease can enjoy tasty, nutritious meals while efficiently controlling their symptoms if they cook and organize their meals with awareness and initiative.

MEAL PLANNING AND RECIPES IN CROHN'S DISEASE

Meal planning and recipe selection for individuals with Crohn's disease should focus on managing symptoms and promoting overall digestive health. Here are some tips and considerations:

Low-Fiber Foods: Crohn's disease can make it difficult to digest high-fiber foods. Opt for low-fiber alternatives such as well-cooked vegetables (without skins), tender fruits (without seeds), white bread, refined grains, and lean proteins.

Soft and Easily Digestible Foods: Incorporate soft, easily digestible foods into your meals, such as soups, stews, smoothies, and cooked grains like rice and oats.

Protein Sources: Choose lean protein sources such as chicken, turkey, fish, eggs, tofu, and well-cooked legumes. These are generally easier to digest compared to fatty or processed meats.

Limit Dairy: Dairy products can be problematic for some individuals with Crohn's disease, especially during flare-ups. Consider dairy alternatives like almond milk, soy milk, or lactose-free products.

Healthy Fats: Include sources of healthy fats in your diet, such as avocado, olive oil, nuts, and seeds. These can help with nutrient absorption and provide essential fatty acids.

Avoid Trigger Foods: Pay attention to foods that trigger your symptoms and avoid them. Common triggers include spicy foods, caffeine, alcohol, and high-fat or fried foods.

Hydration: Stay well-hydrated by drinking plenty of water throughout the day. Avoid sugary drinks and excessive caffeine, as they can worsen digestive symptoms.

Small, Frequent Meals: Instead of large meals, consider eating smaller, more frequent meals throughout the day. This can help manage symptoms like bloating and discomfort.

Cooking Methods: Choose gentle cooking methods such as steaming, boiling, baking, or grilling instead of frying. These methods are easier on the digestive system.

Keep a Food Diary: Keeping track of what you eat and how it affects your symptoms can help identify trigger foods and patterns. This information can guide your meal planning and recipe choices.

Here's a simple recipe idea that aligns with Crohn's disease dietary recommendations:

Chicken and Rice Soup

Ingredients:

- 2 boneless, skinless chicken breasts
- 6 cups low-sodium chicken broth
- 1 cup carrots, diced
- 1 cup celery, diced
- 1 cup white rice
- 2 tablespoons olive oil
- Salt and pepper to taste
- Fresh parsley for garnish (optional)

Instructions:

1. In a large pot, heat olive oil over medium heat. Add diced carrots and

celery and sauté until slightly softened.
2. Add chicken breasts to the pot and season with salt and pepper. Cook until chicken is no longer pink.
3. Pour in chicken broth and bring to a boil. Once boiling, reduce heat to low and simmer for 20-25 minutes until chicken is cooked through.
4. Remove chicken from the pot and shred it using two forks.
5. Return shredded chicken to the pot and add white rice. Simmer for an additional 15-20 minutes until rice is cooked and flavors are well combined.
6. Adjust seasoning if necessary and serve hot, garnished with fresh parsley if desired.

BREAKFAST RECIPES

Banana Oatmeal Smoothie

Ingredients:

- 1 ripe banana
- 1/2 cup rolled oats
- 1 cup almond milk (or any lactose-free milk)
- 1 tablespoon honey or maple syrup (optional)
- Ice cubes (optional)

Instructions:

1. Peel the banana and break it into chunks.
2. In a blender, combine banana chunks, rolled oats, almond milk, and honey or maple syrup (if using).
3. Blend until smooth and creamy.

4. If desired, add ice cubes and blend again until smooth.
5. Pour the smoothie into a glass and enjoy immediately.

Scrambled Eggs with Spinach

Ingredients:

- 2 eggs
- 1 cup fresh spinach leaves, chopped
- 1 tablespoon olive oil
- Salt and pepper to taste

Instructions:

1. In a bowl, whisk the eggs until well beaten. Season with salt and pepper.
2. Heat olive oil in a non-stick skillet over medium heat.
3. Add chopped spinach to the skillet and sauté until wilted.
4. Pour the beaten eggs over the spinach in the skillet.

5. Gently scramble the eggs with a spatula until cooked through.
6. Transfer the scrambled eggs with spinach to a plate and serve hot.

Yogurt Parfait with Berries

Ingredients:

- 1/2 cup lactose-free yogurt (e.g., Greek yogurt)
- 1/4 cup granola (choose a low-fiber option)
- 1/4 cup fresh berries (e.g., strawberries, blueberries, raspberries)

Instructions:

1. In a glass or bowl, layer lactose-free yogurt, granola, and fresh berries.
2. Repeat the layers until all ingredients are used, ending with a layer of berries on top.

3. Serve immediately as a nutritious and refreshing breakfast option.

Peanut Butter Banana Toast

Ingredients:

- 2 slices of white bread (choose low-fiber bread)
- 2 tablespoons peanut butter (choose smooth, creamy peanut butter)
- 1 ripe banana, thinly sliced

Instructions:

1. Toast the slices of bread until golden brown.
2. Spread peanut butter evenly on each slice of toast.
3. Arrange thinly sliced banana on top of the peanut butter.
4. Serve the peanut butter banana toast immediately for a quick and satisfying breakfast.

Rice Porridge with Cinnamon and Applesauce

Ingredients:

- 1/2 cup cooked white rice
- 1/2 cup lactose-free milk or almond milk
- 2 tablespoons unsweetened applesauce
- 1/2 teaspoon ground cinnamon
- 1 teaspoon honey (optional)

Instructions:

1. In a small saucepan, combine cooked white rice and lactose-free milk.
2. Heat the mixture over medium heat, stirring occasionally, until heated through.
3. Stir in unsweetened applesauce and ground cinnamon. Add honey if desired for sweetness.

4. Continue cooking for a few more minutes until the porridge reaches your desired consistency.
5. Transfer the rice porridge to a bowl and serve warm.

LUNCH RECIPES

Baked Chicken and Mashed Potatoes

Ingredients:

- 2 boneless, skinless chicken breasts
- 2 large potatoes, peeled and cubed
- 2 tablespoons olive oil
- Salt and pepper to taste
- 1/4 cup lactose-free milk
- 1 tablespoon unsalted butter (optional)
- Chopped fresh parsley for garnish (optional)

Instructions:

1. Preheat the oven to 375°F (190°C).
2. Place the chicken breasts on a baking sheet lined with parchment paper. Drizzle olive oil over the chicken and season with salt and pepper.
3. Bake the chicken in the preheated oven for 25-30 minutes or until cooked through and no longer pink in the center.
4. While the chicken is baking, boil the cubed potatoes in a pot of salted water until tender, about 15-20 minutes.
5. Drain the cooked potatoes and transfer them to a mixing bowl. Mash the potatoes using a potato masher or fork.
6. Stir in lactose-free milk and unsalted butter (if using) until creamy and smooth.
7. Season the mashed potatoes with salt and pepper to taste.
8. Serve the baked chicken with a side of mashed potatoes, garnished with chopped fresh parsley if desired.

Quinoa Salad with Cucumber and Tomato

Ingredients:

- 1 cup cooked quinoa, cooled
- 1 cucumber, diced
- 1 tomato, diced
- 2 tablespoons chopped fresh parsley
- 2 tablespoons olive oil
- 1 tablespoon lemon juice
- Salt and pepper to taste

Instructions:

1. In a large bowl, combine cooked quinoa, diced cucumber, diced tomato, and chopped fresh parsley.
2. In a small bowl, whisk together olive oil, lemon juice, salt, and pepper to make the dressing.
3. Pour the dressing over the quinoa salad and toss until well combined.

4. Serve the quinoa salad immediately or chill in the refrigerator for 30 minutes before serving to allow the flavors to meld.

Turkey and Cheese Wrap

Ingredients:

- 2 large gluten-free tortillas (or any low-fiber tortillas)
- 4 slices of turkey breast
- 2 slices of low-fat cheese (e.g., Swiss, cheddar)
- 1/2 cup baby spinach leaves
- Mustard or mayonnaise (optional)

Instructions:

1. Lay the tortillas flat on a clean surface.
2. Place two slices of turkey breast on each tortilla.

3. Top each turkey slice with a slice of cheese and a handful of baby spinach leaves.
4. Optionally, spread mustard or mayonnaise over the toppings.
5. Roll up the tortillas tightly to form wraps.
6. Slice each wrap in half diagonally and serve immediately.

Salmon and Avocado Salad

Ingredients:

- 2 (4-ounce) salmon fillets
- 4 cups mixed salad greens
- 1 avocado, sliced
- 1/4 cup cherry tomatoes, halved
- 2 tablespoons olive oil
- 1 tablespoon lemon juice
- Salt and pepper to taste

Instructions:

1. Season the salmon fillets with salt and pepper.
2. Heat olive oil in a non-stick skillet over medium heat.
3. Add the salmon fillets to the skillet and cook for 3-4 minutes per side or until cooked through.
4. In a large bowl, toss mixed salad greens, sliced avocado, and cherry tomatoes with olive oil and lemon juice.
5. Divide the salad mixture between two plates.
6. Place a cooked salmon fillet on top of each salad.
7. Serve the salmon and avocado salad immediately.

Vegetable Stir-Fry with Rice

Ingredients:

- 1 cup cooked white rice
- 1 tablespoon olive oil

- 1 cup mixed vegetables (e.g., bell peppers, broccoli, carrots)
- 2 cloves garlic, minced
- 2 tablespoons low-sodium soy sauce
- 1 teaspoon sesame oil (optional)
- Sesame seeds for garnish (optional)

Instructions:

1. Heat olive oil in a large skillet or wok over medium-high heat.
2. Add mixed vegetables and minced garlic to the skillet. Stir-fry for 3-4 minutes or until vegetables are tender-crisp.
3. Stir in cooked white rice, soy sauce, and sesame oil (if using). Cook for an additional 2-3 minutes, stirring constantly.
4. Transfer the vegetable stir-fry with rice to serving plates.
5. Garnish with sesame seeds if desired and serve hot.

DINNER RECIPES

Baked Salmon with Steamed Vegetables

Ingredients:

- 2 salmon fillets (4-6 ounces each)
- 2 cups mixed vegetables (e.g., carrots, zucchini, bell peppers)
- 2 tablespoons olive oil
- Salt and pepper to taste
- Lemon wedges for serving (optional)

Instructions:

1. Preheat the oven to 375°F (190°C).
2. Place the salmon fillets on a baking sheet lined with parchment paper.
3. Drizzle olive oil over the salmon fillets and season with salt and pepper.
4. Bake the salmon in the preheated oven for 12-15 minutes or until cooked through and flakes easily with a fork.

5. While the salmon is baking, steam the mixed vegetables until tender.
6. Serve the baked salmon with steamed vegetables on the side.
7. Squeeze fresh lemon juice over the salmon before serving, if desired.

Turkey and Vegetable Stir-Fry

Ingredients:

- 1 pound ground turkey
- 2 cups mixed vegetables (e.g., broccoli, bell peppers, snap peas)
- 2 tablespoons olive oil
- 2 cloves garlic, minced
- 2 tablespoons low-sodium soy sauce
- 1 teaspoon sesame oil (optional)
- Cooked white rice for serving

Instructions:

1. Heat olive oil in a large skillet or wok over medium-high heat.
2. Add ground turkey to the skillet and cook until browned, breaking it apart with a spoon.
3. Add mixed vegetables and minced garlic to the skillet. Stir-fry for 5-7 minutes or until vegetables are tender-crisp.
4. Stir in low-sodium soy sauce and sesame oil (if using). Cook for an additional 2-3 minutes, stirring constantly.
5. Serve the turkey and vegetable stir-fry over cooked white rice.

Chicken and Rice Casserole

Ingredients:

- 2 boneless, skinless chicken breasts, cooked and shredded
- 2 cups cooked white rice

- 1 cup mixed vegetables (e.g., peas, carrots, corn)
- 1 cup lactose-free or low-lactose cream of chicken soup
- 1/2 cup shredded cheddar cheese (optional)
- Salt and pepper to taste

Instructions:

1. Preheat the oven to 350°F (175°C).
2. In a large mixing bowl, combine shredded chicken, cooked white rice, mixed vegetables, and cream of chicken soup. Mix well to combine.
3. Season the mixture with salt and pepper to taste.
4. Transfer the mixture to a greased baking dish.
5. Sprinkle shredded cheddar cheese over the top, if using.
6. Bake the chicken and rice casserole in the preheated oven for 25-30 minutes or until bubbly and heated through.

7. Serve hot as a comforting and satisfying dinner option.

Spinach and Feta Stuffed Chicken Breast

Ingredients:

- 2 boneless, skinless chicken breasts
- 1 cup fresh spinach leaves
- 1/4 cup crumbled feta cheese
- 1 tablespoon olive oil
- Salt and pepper to taste
- Toothpicks

Instructions:

1. Preheat the oven to 375°F (190°C).
2. Using a sharp knife, make a horizontal slit along the side of each chicken breast to create a pocket.
3. Stuff each chicken breast with fresh spinach leaves and crumbled feta cheese.

4. Secure the openings of the chicken breasts with toothpicks to hold the stuffing in place.
5. Season the stuffed chicken breasts with salt and pepper.
6. Heat olive oil in an oven-safe skillet over medium-high heat.
7. Add the stuffed chicken breasts to the skillet and sear for 2-3 minutes on each side until golden brown.
8. Transfer the skillet to the preheated oven and bake for 20-25 minutes or until the chicken is cooked through and reaches an internal temperature of 165°F (75°C).
9. Remove the toothpicks before serving.

Turkey and Rice Soup

Ingredients:

- 1 tablespoon olive oil
- 1 pound ground turkey
- 1 onion, diced

- 2 carrots, diced
- 2 celery stalks, diced
- 6 cups low-sodium chicken broth
- 1 cup cooked white rice
- Salt and pepper to taste
- Chopped fresh parsley for garnish (optional)

Instructions:

1. Heat olive oil in a large pot over medium heat.
2. Add ground turkey to the pot and cook until browned, breaking it apart with a spoon.
3. Add diced onion, carrots, and celery to the pot. Cook for 5-7 minutes or until vegetables are softened.
4. Pour in low-sodium chicken broth and bring to a simmer.
5. Stir in cooked white rice and season the soup with salt and pepper to taste.

6. Simmer the turkey and rice soup for 15-20 minutes to allow the flavors to meld.
7. Ladle the soup into bowls and garnish with chopped fresh parsley, if desired.
8. Serve hot as a comforting and nourishing dinner option.

DESSERT AND SNACK RECIPES

Peanut Butter Banana Bites

Ingredients:

- 2 ripe bananas
- 2 tablespoons peanut butter (smooth, creamy)
- 2 tablespoons dark chocolate chips (optional)

Instructions:

1. Peel the bananas and cut them into slices, about 1/2 inch thick.
2. Spread peanut butter on half of the banana slices.
3. Top each peanut butter-covered banana slice with another banana slice to form sandwiches.
4. Optionally, melt dark chocolate chips in the microwave or on the stove.
5. Drizzle melted chocolate over the banana sandwiches or dip each sandwich halfway into the melted chocolate.
6. Place the peanut butter banana bites on a baking sheet lined with parchment paper.
7. Freeze for 1-2 hours or until the chocolate sets.
8. Serve chilled as a delicious and satisfying snack or dessert.

Greek Yogurt with Honey and Berries

Ingredients:

- 1 cup lactose-free Greek yogurt
- 2 tablespoons honey (or maple syrup)
- 1/2 cup fresh berries (e.g., strawberries, blueberries, raspberries)

Instructions:

1. In a bowl, spoon Greek yogurt.
2. Drizzle honey (or maple syrup) over the yogurt.
3. Top with fresh berries.
4. Serve immediately as a nutritious and refreshing snack or dessert.

Rice Cake with Almond Butter and Banana

Ingredients:

- 1 rice cake
- 1 tablespoon almond butter (or any nut butter)
- 1/2 banana, thinly sliced

- Cinnamon (optional)

Instructions:

1. Spread almond butter evenly on the rice cake.
2. Arrange thinly sliced banana on top of the almond butter.
3. Optionally, sprinkle cinnamon over the banana slices for extra flavor.
4. Serve the rice cake with almond butter and banana as a quick and satisfying snack.

Trail Mix with Nuts and Dried Fruit

Ingredients:

- 1/4 cup almonds, unsalted
- 1/4 cup walnuts, unsalted
- 1/4 cup pumpkin seeds
- 1/4 cup dried cranberries
- 1/4 cup dried apricots, chopped

Instructions:

1. In a bowl, combine almonds, walnuts, pumpkin seeds, dried cranberries, and chopped dried apricots.
2. Mix well to distribute ingredients evenly.
3. Portion the trail mix into individual snack-sized bags or containers for convenient grab-and-go snacks.

Cottage Cheese with Pineapple Slices

Ingredients:

- 1/2 cup lactose-free cottage cheese
- 1/2 cup fresh pineapple slices (or canned pineapple in juice)

Instructions:

1. Spoon cottage cheese into a bowl.
2. Top with fresh pineapple slices.

3. Serve chilled as a simple and satisfying snack or dessert option.

APPETIZERS RECIPES

Caprese Skewers

Ingredients:

- Cherry tomatoes
- Fresh mozzarella balls
- Fresh basil leaves
- Balsamic glaze (store-bought or homemade*)

Instructions:

1. Assemble the skewers by threading one cherry tomato, one mozzarella ball, and one basil leaf onto each skewer.
2. Arrange the caprese skewers on a serving platter.

3. Drizzle balsamic glaze over the skewers just before serving.
4. Serve immediately as a light and refreshing appetizer.

Cucumber Hummus Bites

Ingredients:

- Cucumber, sliced into rounds
- Hummus (store-bought or homemade*)
- Cherry tomatoes, halved
- Fresh parsley or dill for garnish (optional)

Instructions:

1. Place cucumber slices on a serving platter.
2. Top each cucumber slice with a small dollop of hummus.
3. Garnish with a halved cherry tomato and fresh parsley or dill, if desired.

4. Serve the cucumber hummus bites chilled as a crunchy and flavorful appetizer.

Greek Salad Skewers

Ingredients:

- Cucumber, cut into cubes
- Cherry tomatoes
- Kalamata olives, pitted
- Feta cheese, cut into cubes
- Fresh parsley or oregano for garnish (optional)
- Greek salad dressing (store-bought or homemade*)

Instructions:

1. Assemble the skewers by threading cucumber cubes, cherry tomatoes, kalamata olives, and feta cheese cubes onto each skewer.

2. Arrange the Greek salad skewers on a serving platter.
3. Drizzle Greek salad dressing over the skewers just before serving.
4. Garnish with fresh parsley or oregano, if desired.
5. Serve immediately as a flavorful and colorful appetizer option.

Stuffed Mini Bell Peppers

Ingredients:

- Mini bell peppers, halved and seeds removed
- Cream cheese (regular or lactose-free)
- Green onions, chopped
- Paprika for garnish (optional)

Instructions:

1. Preheat the oven to 375°F (190°C).
2. In a mixing bowl, combine cream cheese and chopped green onions.

3. Spoon the cream cheese mixture into each halved mini bell pepper.
4. Arrange the stuffed mini bell peppers on a baking sheet lined with parchment paper.
5. Sprinkle paprika over the stuffed peppers for additional flavor, if desired.
6. Bake in the preheated oven for 10-12 minutes or until the peppers are tender and the filling is heated through.
7. Serve the stuffed mini bell peppers warm as a savory appetizer option.

Smoked Salmon Cucumber Bites

Ingredients:

- English cucumber, sliced into rounds
- Smoked salmon slices
- Cream cheese (regular or lactose-free)
- Fresh dill for garnish

Instructions:

1. Place cucumber slices on a serving platter.
2. Spread a thin layer of cream cheese on each cucumber slice.
3. Top with a piece of smoked salmon.
4. Garnish with fresh dill.
5. Serve the smoked salmon cucumber bites chilled as an elegant and flavorful appetizer.

HEALTHY RECIPES

Quinoa Salad with Lemon-Herb Dressing

Ingredients:

- 1 cup quinoa, rinsed
- 2 cups water or low-sodium vegetable broth
- 1 cucumber, diced
- 1 bell pepper, diced
- 1/4 cup red onion, finely chopped

- 1/4 cup fresh parsley, chopped
- Juice of 1 lemon
- 2 tablespoons olive oil
- 1 teaspoon dried oregano
- Salt and pepper to taste

Instructions:

1. In a medium saucepan, bring water or vegetable broth to a boil.
2. Add quinoa, reduce heat to low, cover, and simmer for 15-20 minutes or until quinoa is cooked and liquid is absorbed.
3. Fluff cooked quinoa with a fork and let it cool to room temperature.
4. In a large mixing bowl, combine cooked quinoa, diced cucumber, diced bell pepper, chopped red onion, and chopped parsley.
5. In a small bowl, whisk together lemon juice, olive oil, dried oregano, salt, and pepper to make the dressing.

6. Pour the dressing over the quinoa salad and toss until well combined.
7. Adjust seasoning if necessary.
8. Serve the quinoa salad chilled or at room temperature as a nutritious and satisfying meal.

Baked Chicken and Vegetables

Ingredients:

- 2 boneless, skinless chicken breasts
- 2 cups mixed vegetables (e.g., broccoli, carrots, cauliflower)
- 2 tablespoons olive oil
- 1 teaspoon garlic powder
- 1 teaspoon dried thyme
- Salt and pepper to taste

Instructions:

1. Preheat the oven to 400°F (200°C).

2. Place chicken breasts and mixed vegetables on a baking sheet lined with parchment paper.
3. Drizzle olive oil over the chicken and vegetables.
4. Sprinkle garlic powder, dried thyme, salt, and pepper evenly over the chicken and vegetables.
5. Bake in the preheated oven for 20-25 minutes or until the chicken is cooked through and vegetables are tender.
6. Remove from the oven and let it rest for a few minutes before serving.
7. Serve the baked chicken and vegetables hot as a balanced and wholesome meal.

Turkey and Quinoa Stuffed Peppers

Ingredients:

- 4 bell peppers, halved and seeds removed
- 1 cup cooked quinoa

- 1 pound lean ground turkey
- 1 small onion, diced
- 1 garlic clove, minced
- 1 teaspoon dried basil
- 1 teaspoon dried oregano
- Salt and pepper to taste
- 1 cup tomato sauce

Instructions:

1. Preheat the oven to 375°F (190°C).
2. In a large skillet, cook ground turkey over medium heat until browned.
3. Add diced onion and minced garlic to the skillet and cook until softened.
4. Stir in cooked quinoa, dried basil, dried oregano, salt, and pepper. Cook for another 2-3 minutes.
5. Spoon the turkey-quinoa mixture into each halved bell pepper.
6. Place stuffed peppers in a baking dish and pour tomato sauce over them.
7. Cover the baking dish with aluminum foil and bake in the preheated oven for

30-35 minutes or until peppers are tender.
8. Remove the foil and bake for an additional 5-10 minutes.
9. Serve the turkey and quinoa stuffed peppers hot as a flavorful and nutritious meal.

Veggie and Bean Soup

Ingredients:

- 1 tablespoon olive oil
- 1 onion, diced
- 2 carrots, diced
- 2 celery stalks, diced
- 2 cloves garlic, minced
- 1 teaspoon dried thyme
- 1 teaspoon dried rosemary
- 4 cups low-sodium vegetable broth
- 1 can (15 ounces) cannellini beans, drained and rinsed
- 1 cup chopped kale or spinach
- Salt and pepper to taste

Instructions:

1. Heat olive oil in a large pot over medium heat.
2. Add diced onion, carrots, and celery to the pot. Cook until vegetables are softened.
3. Stir in minced garlic, dried thyme, and dried rosemary. Cook for another minute.
4. Pour vegetable broth into the pot and bring to a simmer.
5. Add cannellini beans and chopped kale or spinach. Simmer for 10-15 minutes.
6. Season with salt and pepper to taste.
7. Serve the veggie and bean soup hot as a comforting and nourishing meal.

Lentil Salad with Lemon-Tahini Dressing

Ingredients:

- 1 cup dried green lentils

- 2 cups water
- 1 cucumber, diced
- 1 bell pepper, diced
- 1/4 cup red onion, finely chopped
- 1/4 cup fresh parsley, chopped
- Juice of 1 lemon
- 2 tablespoons tahini
- 1 garlic clove, minced
- Salt and pepper to taste

Instructions:

1. Rinse lentils under cold water and drain.
2. In a medium saucepan, combine lentils and water. Bring to a boil, then reduce heat to low and simmer for 20-25 minutes or until lentils are tender.
3. Drain any excess water from the cooked lentils and let them cool to room temperature.
4. In a large mixing bowl, combine cooked lentils, diced cucumber, diced

bell pepper, chopped red onion, and chopped parsley.
5. In a small bowl, whisk together lemon juice, tahini, minced garlic, salt, and pepper to make the dressing.
6. Pour the dressing over the lentil salad and toss until well combined.
7. Adjust seasoning if necessary.
8. Serve the lentil salad chilled or at room temperature as a nutritious and flavorful meal.

28DAY MEAL PLAN

Day 1:

Breakfast: Banana Oatmeal Smoothie

- 1 ripe banana
- 1/2 cup rolled oats
- 1 cup almond milk (or any lactose-free milk)

- 1 tablespoon honey or maple syrup (optional)

Lunch: Greek Salad Skewers

- Cucumber, cherry tomatoes, kalamata olives, feta cheese
- Greek salad dressing (store-bought or homemade)

Snack: Rice Cake with Almond Butter and Banana

Dinner: Baked Salmon with Steamed Vegetables

- 2 salmon fillets
- Mixed vegetables (e.g., broccoli, carrots, cauliflower)
- Olive oil, garlic powder, dried thyme, salt, and pepper

Day 2:

Breakfast: Greek Yogurt with Honey and Berries

- 1 cup lactose-free Greek yogurt
- 2 tablespoons honey (or maple syrup)
- 1/2 cup fresh berries (e.g., strawberries, blueberries, raspberries)

Lunch: Turkey and Quinoa Stuffed Peppers

- Bell peppers, ground turkey, cooked quinoa, onion, garlic, herbs, tomato sauce

Snack: Cottage Cheese with Pineapple Slices

Dinner: Vegetable Stir-Fry with Rice

- Mixed vegetables (e.g., bell peppers, broccoli, carrots)

- Cooked white rice
- Olive oil, garlic, low-sodium soy sauce

Day 3:

Breakfast: Peanut Butter Banana Bites

- Ripe bananas, peanut butter, dark chocolate chips (optional)

Lunch: Lentil Salad with Lemon-Tahini Dressing

- Dried green lentils, cucumber, bell pepper, red onion, fresh parsley, lemon, tahini, garlic

Snack: Trail Mix with Nuts and Dried Fruit

Dinner: Chicken and Rice Casserole

- Boneless, skinless chicken breasts, cooked white rice, mixed vegetables, cream of chicken soup, shredded cheddar cheese (optional)

Day 4:

Breakfast: Quinoa Salad with Lemon-Herb Dressing

- Quinoa, cucumber, bell pepper, red onion, fresh parsley, lemon, olive oil, dried herbs

Lunch: Turkey and Bean Soup

- Ground turkey, mixed vegetables, low-sodium vegetable broth, cannellini beans, kale or spinach, herbs

Snack: Stuffed Mini Bell Peppers

- Mini bell peppers, cream cheese, green onions, paprika

Dinner: Veggie and Bean Soup

- Onion, carrots, celery, garlic, dried herbs, low-sodium vegetable broth, cannellini beans, kale or spinach

Day 5:

Breakfast: Cucumber Hummus Bites

- Cucumber, hummus, cherry tomatoes, fresh parsley or dill

Lunch: Spinach and Feta Stuffed Chicken Breast

- Boneless, skinless chicken breasts, fresh spinach leaves, feta cheese, olive oil, salt, and pepper

Snack: Greek Salad Skewers

Dinner: Baked Chicken and Vegetables

- Boneless, skinless chicken breasts, mixed vegetables, olive oil, garlic powder, dried thyme, salt, and pepper

Day 6:

Breakfast: Rice Porridge with Cinnamon and Applesauce

- Cooked white rice, lactose-free milk, unsweetened applesauce, cinnamon, honey (optional)

Lunch: Chicken and Vegetable Stir-Fry

- Chicken breast, mixed vegetables, olive oil, low-sodium soy sauce

Snack: Smoked Salmon Cucumber Bites

- English cucumber, smoked salmon, cream cheese, fresh dill

Dinner: Quinoa Salad with Lemon-Herb Dressing

Day 7:

Breakfast: Yogurt Parfait with Berries

- Lactose-free yogurt, granola, fresh berries

Lunch: Vegetable Stir-Fry with Rice

Snack: Peanut Butter Banana Toast

- White bread, peanut butter, ripe banana

Dinner: Turkey and Rice Soup

- Ground turkey, onion, carrots, celery, low-sodium chicken broth, cooked white rice

Day 8:

Breakfast: Banana Oatmeal Smoothie

Lunch: Lentil Soup

- Dried green lentils, carrot, celery, onion, garlic, low-sodium vegetable broth, herbs

Snack: Greek Yogurt with Honey and Berries

Dinner: Grilled Chicken Breast with Steamed Asparagus

- Chicken breast, asparagus, olive oil, lemon, salt, and pepper

Day 9:

Breakfast: Peanut Butter Banana Bites

Lunch: Turkey and Quinoa Stuffed Peppers

Snack: Rice Cake with Almond Butter and Banana

Dinner: Baked Salmon with Lemon-Dill Sauce

- Salmon fillet, lemon, fresh dill, olive oil, salt, and pepper

Day 10:

Breakfast: Quinoa Salad with Lemon-Herb Dressing

Lunch: Chicken and Vegetable Stir-Fry

Snack: Cottage Cheese with Pineapple Slices

Dinner: Veggie and Bean Soup

Day 11:

Breakfast: Cucumber Hummus Bites

Lunch: Spinach and Feta Stuffed Chicken Breast

Snack: Greek Salad Skewers

Dinner: Baked Chicken and Vegetables

Day 12:

Breakfast: Greek Yogurt with Honey and Berries

Lunch: Lentil Salad with Lemon-Tahini Dressing

Snack: Stuffed Mini Bell Peppers

Dinner: Turkey and Rice Soup

Day 13:

Breakfast: Rice Porridge with Cinnamon and Applesauce

Lunch: Caprese Skewers

Snack: Smoked Salmon Cucumber Bites

Dinner: Quinoa Salad with Lemon-Herb Dressing

Day 14:

Breakfast: Yogurt Parfait with Berries

Lunch: Greek Salad with Grilled Chicken

- Mixed greens, cucumber, cherry tomatoes, olives, feta cheese, grilled chicken breast, Greek salad dressing

Snack: Peanut Butter Banana Toast

Dinner: Veggie and Bean Chili

- Mixed vegetables, beans (e.g., kidney beans, black beans), diced tomatoes, vegetable broth, chili powder, cumin, garlic powder

Day 15:

Breakfast: Banana Oatmeal Smoothie

Lunch: Lentil Soup

Snack: Greek Yogurt with Honey and Berries

Dinner: Grilled Chicken Breast with Steamed Asparagus

Day 16:

Breakfast: Peanut Butter Banana Bites

Lunch: Turkey and Quinoa Stuffed Peppers

Snack: Rice Cake with Almond Butter and Banana

Dinner: Baked Salmon with Lemon-Dill Sauce

Day 17:

Breakfast: Quinoa Salad with Lemon-Herb Dressing

Lunch: Chicken and Vegetable Stir-Fry

Snack: Cottage Cheese with Pineapple Slices

Dinner: Veggie and Bean Soup

Day 18:

Breakfast: Cucumber Hummus Bites

Lunch: Spinach and Feta Stuffed Chicken Breast

Snack: Greek Salad Skewers

Dinner: Baked Chicken and Vegetables

Day 19:

Breakfast: Greek Yogurt with Honey and Berries

Lunch: Lentil Salad with Lemon-Tahini Dressing

Snack: Stuffed Mini Bell Peppers

Dinner: Turkey and Rice Soup

Day 20:

Breakfast: Rice Porridge with Cinnamon and Applesauce

Lunch: Caprese Skewers

Snack: Smoked Salmon Cucumber Bites

Dinner: Quinoa Salad with Lemon-Herb Dressing

Day 21:

Breakfast: Yogurt Parfait with Berries

Lunch: Greek Salad with Grilled Chicken

Snack: Peanut Butter Banana Toast

Dinner: Veggie and Bean Chili

Day 22:

Breakfast: Banana Oatmeal Smoothie

Lunch: Lentil Soup

Snack: Greek Yogurt with Honey and Berries

Dinner: Grilled Chicken Breast with Steamed Asparagus

Day 23:

Breakfast: Peanut Butter Banana Bites

Lunch: Turkey and Quinoa Stuffed Peppers

Snack: Rice Cake with Almond Butter and Banana

Dinner: Baked Salmon with Lemon-Dill Sauce

Day 24:

Breakfast: Quinoa Salad with Lemon-Herb Dressing

Lunch: Chicken and Vegetable Stir-Fry

Snack: Cottage Cheese with Pineapple Slices

Dinner: Veggie and Bean Soup

Day 25:

Breakfast: Cucumber Hummus Bites

Lunch: Spinach and Feta Stuffed Chicken Breast

Snack: Greek Salad Skewers

Dinner: Baked Chicken and Vegetables

Day 26:

Breakfast: Greek Yogurt with Honey and Berries

Lunch: Lentil Salad with Lemon-Tahini Dressing

Snack: Stuffed Mini Bell Peppers

Dinner: Turkey and Rice Soup

Day 27:

Breakfast: Rice Porridge with Cinnamon and Applesauce

Lunch: Caprese Skewers

Snack: Smoked Salmon Cucumber Bites

Dinner: Quinoa Salad with Lemon-Herb Dressing

Day 28:

Breakfast: Yogurt Parfait with Berries

Lunch: Greek Salad with Grilled Chicken

Snack: Peanut Butter Banana Toast

Dinner: Veggie and Bean Chili

CONCLUSION

Congratulations on taking the first step towards healing and managing your Crohn's disease! This cookbook has provided you with the tools and recipes to transform your diet and improve your overall health. Remember, every small change adds up, and with these quick and easy recipes, you'll be on your way to a happier, healthier you in no time!

Don't let Crohn's disease hold you back - take control of your diet and your life. With the 30-Minute Solution Crohn's Disease Diet Cookbook for Beginners, you'll be enjoying delicious, nutritious meals in no time. Happy cooking and happy healing!"

This conclusion aims to:

- Encourage and congratulate the reader on taking the first step towards managing their Crohn's disease
- Emphasize the importance of small changes adding up to make a big difference
- Encourage the reader to take control of their diet and life

- End with a positive and uplifting note, wishing the reader happy cooking and happy healing.

THE END

www.ingramcontent.com/pod-product-compliance
Lightning Source LLC
Chambersburg PA
CBHW071212240526
45470CB00018B/1795